Accident and Emergency Medicine

David G. Ferguson MB BCh BAO FRCS(Ed) FFAFM
Director of Emergency Services,
Royal Hallamshire Hospital, Sheffield, UK
Honorary Lecturer in Accident and Emergency Medicine,
University of Sheffield

David I. Fodden MB ChB FRCS(Ed) DA(UK) FFAEM
Consultant in Accident and Emergency Medicine,
Pinderfields General Hospital
Wakefield, UK

SECOND EDITION

CHURCHILL
LIVINGSTONE

EDINBURGH LONDON NE
SAN FRANCISCO SYDNEY TORONTO 1998

CHURCHILL LIVINGSTONE
A Division of Harcourt Brace and Company
Limited.

© Longman Group UK Limited 1993
Harcourt Brace Company Limited 1998

◢▶ is a registered trademark of Harcourt Brace
and Company Limited.

First published as Colour Guide: Accident and
Emergency Medicine 1993
Second Colour Guide edition 1998

ISBN 0 443 06029 0

British Library Cataloguing in Publication Data
A catalogue record for this book is available from
the British Library.

Library of Congress Cataloging in Publication Data
A catalog record for this book is available from
the Library of Congress.

Medical knowledge is constantly
changing. As new information
becomes available, changes in
treatment, procedures, equipment
and the use of drugs become
necessary. The editors/authors/
contributors and the publishers
have, as far as it is possible,
taken care to ensure that the
information given in this text is
accurate and up to date.
However, readers are strongly
advised to confirm that the
information, especially with
regard to drug usage, complies
with current legislation and
standards of practice.

The
publisher's
policy is to use
**paper manufactured
from sustainable forests**

Produced by Addison Wesley
Longman China Limited, Hong Kong.
SWTC/01

For Churchill Livingstone

Publisher: Timothy Horne
Project editor: James Dale
Project controller: Nancy Arnott
Design direction: Erik Bigland

Acknowledgements

Most slide collections are built up over many years by swapping interesting and classical cases with colleagues. The following are those whom we know have allowed us to use their own slides, but we fully acknowledge those other, unnamed colleagues, from whom we have built up our own collection over the years. We would like to thank the Resuscitation Council (UK) for their help and permission to use the new 1997 Resuscitation Guidelines for use in the United Kingdom.

- Resuscitation Council (UK)   Figures 11, 15
- Mr IG Rennie   Figures 33, 35, 36, 37, 39
- Mr S Ward   Figures 41, 42
- Mr PD Bull   Figures 61
- Dr NA Barrington   Figures 63, 64, 72, 73, 122
- Mr WEG Thomas   Figure 102
- Dr D Harris   Figure 103
- Dr GR Kinghorn   Figures 110, 111
- Dr CI Harrington   Figures 147, 200
- Dr JK Gosnold   Figures 192, 193, 194
- Professor DR Triger   Figure 198

Sheffield   D.G.F.
1998   D.I.F.

To our medical students
'Your see but you do not observe.'
The memoirs of Sherlock Holmes
The Crooked Man

The creator of Sherlock Holmes, Sir Arthur Conan Doyle, was as a medical student inspired by his teacher, Mr Joseph Bell, a surgeon at the Royal Infirmary, Edinburgh, and a President of the Royal College of Surgeons of Edinburgh. Sir Arthur learned the great value of true observation which enables clinicians to glean essential general information about their patients, as well as their clinical conditions.

Sheffield   D.G.F.
1998   D.I.F.

Contents

1 / The Accident and Emergency department

The patient and the A & E team

The Accident and Emergency (A & E) department is the front door of every hospital and through it will come all manner of injuries and illnesses. It is difficult to define exactly who should be seen in the unit: it could be stated that anyone with an injury more than 24 h old should not be seen and staff often feel that patients who have self-referred have inappropriate and trivial conditions which would be better seen by their general practitioners.

The patient

The A & E department offers an ever open door which can act as a fail-safe mechanism for the community and ensures that anyone requiring emergency treatment can always be afforded it. Remember that the public do not have the knowledge of the doctors and nurses in the A & E department and, because of this, things which seem trivial to us may appear very serious to them.

Figure 1 shows a breakdown of patients presenting to a selection of A & E departments. The majority of patients are 'walking wounded', and a large proportion of the stretcher cases have an acute medical disorder. Between 20 and 25% of patients fall into the paediatric age group.

The team

The A & E department has a large team (Fig. 2) of staff who work closely with the community through general practitioners and the ambulance service. Within the department, because of the nature of the work and, in particular, because of the emergency and stressful situations that can arise, it is essential that everyone works as a team. Domestics, porters, ECG technicians, social workers, secretaries, reception staff, doctors and nurses all form part of the team and no one individual is more important than another.

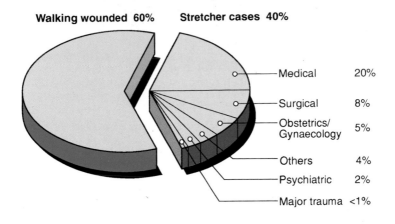

Walking wounded 60%　　**Stretcher cases 40%**

Medical	20%
Surgical	8%
Obstetrics/ Gynaecology	5%
Others	4%
Psychiatric	2%
Major trauma	<1%

Fig. 1 A breakdown of patients presenting to a selection of A & E departments.

Fig. 2 The A & E team.

The workload

The workload of an A & E department can broadly be divided into major (trolley) cases and minor (walking wounded) cases.

Major cases

Those conditions presenting to the trolley area may require resuscitation, and generally consist of serious medical and surgical conditions (Fig. 3). Major trauma is not common and the majority of the workload consists of acute medical emergencies. With the improved medical and social care in the community, there are more elderly cases coming to hospital and the average age of those being seen is now greater than that a few years ago. This creates bed management problems as the elderly often require prolonged rehabilitation.

Minor cases

The area catering for walking wounded deals with sprains, strains, minor fractures and wounds (Fig. 4). The biggest problem with this work is that it tends to be very repetitive and there is a great temptation to be less careful when examining and documenting such cases. The majority of litigation against A & E departments stems from such errors.

There is a wealth of pathology in this area, if the staff are astute enough to note it, even though it may not be related directly to the presenting complaint. This is an excellent area to learn to work quickly and efficiently.

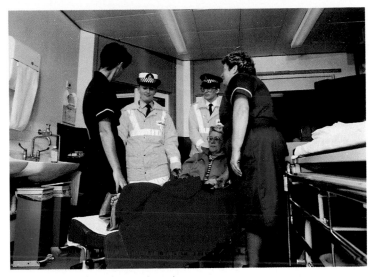

Fig. 3 Reception of a patient on the majors area.

Fig. 4 A case in the minors area.

Resuscitation (1)

General points

The management of a cardiorespiratory arrest is something which demands smooth, efficient teamwork (Fig. 5) between medical, nursing and paramedical staff if a successful outcome is to be achieved. It is essential that the team is familiar with the equipment to be used (Figs 6 & 7), and that it is checked on a daily basis. Frequent rehearsals using manikins and critical self-audits are necessary, as are adequate numbers of staff. Each team member should have a clearly defined role and one should be elected as team leader. All major decisions should be directed through this person, and he/she should not take any active role in the resuscitation. The Resuscitation Council (UK) have produced guidelines for the management of resuscitation situations (Fig. 11, see p. 10, and Fig. 15, see p. 14), and all medical and nursing personnel must be fully familiar with these.

The relatives

In the event of an unsuccessful resuscitation, it is important to consider the relatives. They should be told in simple words what has happened and what resuscitative efforts were made. It is normal practice in England for the Coroner to be informed of all A & E deaths, and this should be explained as a routine procedure to the relatives. Although a post mortem examination may be ordered, it is not uncommon for the General Practitioner to be willing to sign a Death Certificate if the patient has been seen recently and they are happy that the cause of death was likely to have been due to some serious previously diagnosed condition, such as ischaemic heart disease.

Fig. 5 The resuscitation team at work.

Fig. 6 Defibrillator with gel pads.

Fig. 7 Necessary airway equipment for resuscitation.

Resuscitation (2)

Adult basic life support

This skill should be as widely taught as possible, as early effective BLS will greatly improve the chances of survival for both cardiac and non cardiac cases of arrest. No equipment is required, only knowledge and practice.

1. Ensure safety of the rescuer and the victim.
2. Check the victim for responsiveness, a gentle shake and ask loudly 'Are you alright?'
3. If no response, shout for help.

   Open the airway by tilting the head and doing a chin lift.

   Do not do the head tilt if there is any question of neck trauma. Check for breathing, look, listen and feel for up to 10 seconds. If there is no breathing, pinch the nose and put your mouth over the victim's mouth and give two effective rescue breaths, watching the chest rise and fall (Fig. 8).
4. Assess for signs of circulation by feeling the carotid pulse, do not take more than 10 seconds to do this. If no circulation, start chest compression. The heel of the hands should be over the middle of the lower half of the sternum (Fig. 9), and the sternum should be depressed 4–5 cm on compression. Do 15 compressions at the approximate rate of 100 per min (Fig. 10).
5. If no circulation, continue mouth to mouth with two rescue breaths and follow this with 15 chest compressions. Check the circulation every minute.
6. If there are two rescuers, then one can do the rescue breaths and the other the chest compressions: the ratio is 1 breath to 5 compressions.

Fig. 8 Mouth to mouth resuscitation.

Fig. 9 Identifying the correct position for the hands on the sternum.

Fig. 10 External cardiac massage.

Resuscitation (3)

When do you go for help if you are on your own?
If the likely cause of unconsciousness is trauma or drowning, or if the victim is an infant or child, resuscitate for 1 min and then go for help.

If the victim is an adult, and the cause of unconsciousness is not trauma or drowning, assume the probable cause is cardiac. Assuming that you have determined unresponsiveness and absence of breathing, go for help.

Most adults who can be saved from cardiac arrest are individuals who are in ventricular fibrillation or pulseless ventricular tachycardia. Electrical defibrillation provides the single most important therapy for the treatment of these patients.

Resuscitation Council (UK)

Adult Basic Life Support

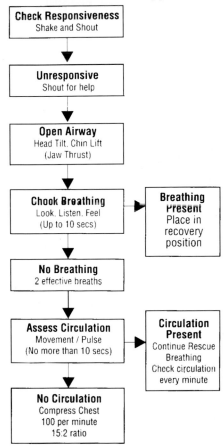

Send or go for assistance as soon as possible according to guidelines

Fig. 11 Adult Basic Life Support Guidelines (1997 Resuscitation Council (UK) Guidelines for use in the United Kingdom).

Resuscitation (4)

Adult advanced life support

1. This is the natural follow on from basic life support, and occurs with the arrival of a monitor/defibrillator.
2. If the collapse was initially witnessed, a precordial thump can be administered prior to the attachment of the monitor/defibrillator.
3. With the attachment of the monitor/defibrillator, assess the rhythm and check for a pulse.

VF/Pulseless VT

These are the most common primary arrhythmias causing cardiac arrest (Figs 12 & 13). The majority of eventual survivors will come from this group. The chances of success with defibrillation declines by about 5% with each minute's delay. Even the best quality BLS can only slow this process.

1. Place one defibrillator paddle below the right clavicle and to the side of the sternum. The other paddle is placed outside the position of the normal cardiac apex (Fig. 16, see p. 16). Ensure you use gel pads or an appropriate contact gel to decrease the skin resistance and prevent burning.
2. Instruct everybody to stand clear and defibrillate at 200 joules. If there is a rhythm compatible with a cardiac output, check the pulse.
   There can be a delay in the rhythm trace settling down after defibrillation and although there may be an appropriate rhythm, the myocardial contractions can initially be weak, making it difficult to feel a pulse. If no response, give a further 200 joule shock, and if no rhythm change, follow this with a 360 joule shock.
3. Do 1 min CPR: secure the airway and gain intravenous access and give 1 mg of Epinephrine intravenously.
4. Consider other potentially reversible causes of VF/VT.
5. If VF/VT persists, continue the cycle up to three defibrillation discharges at 360 joules each, followed by a 1 min CPR, give 1 mg of Epinephrine every 3 min (this will approximately correlate with the time taken to carry out the full cycle). Check for a pulse if there is a rhythm change compatible with a cardiac output.
6. Persist while the patient is in VF/VT.

Fig. 12 Ventricular tachycardia.

Fig. 13 Ventricular fibrillation.

Fig. 14 The undulating line of asystole.

Resuscitation (5)

Non-VF/VT

These patients may have asystole (Fig. 14, see p. 12), (pulseless electrical activity) or PEA
these rhythms tend to have a less favourable prognosis, but there are some situations where they can be caused by reversible conditions.

The Four Hs

Hypoxia
Hypovolaemia
Hyper/hypokalaemia and metabolic disorders
Hypothermia

The Four Ts

Tension pneumothorax
Tamponade
Toxic/therapeutic disturbances
Thromboembolic/mechanical obstruction

Three mins CPR: secure airway and gain venous access. Epinephrine is given every 3 min. Use other drug therapies as appropriate, e.g. Atropine. If a rhythm compatible with a cardiac output is present, do a pulse check. If VF/VT occurs, then follow the left hand path of the algorithm (Fig. 15). If the patient remains in a non-VF/VT rhthym, continue to follow the right hand path of the algorithm for as long as is considered appropriate.

Resuscitation Council (UK)

CARDIAC ARREST

```
        ┌─────────────────────┐
        │    BLS Algorithm    │
        │    if appropriate   │
        └─────────────────────┘
                  │
        ┌─────────────────────┐
        │   Precordial Thump  │
        │    if appropriate   │
        └─────────────────────┘
                  │
        ┌─────────────────────┐
        │       Attach        │
        │ Defibrillator/Monitor│
        └─────────────────────┘
                  │
          ◆ Assess Rhythm ◆
        ┌─────────────────────┐
        │    ± Check Pulse    │
        └─────────────────────┘
```

VF/VT   **Non VF/VT**

┌──────────────────┐   ┌─────────────────────────────────┐   ┌──────────────┐
│ Defibrillate x 3 │   │   During CPR   │   │   │
│ as necessary   │   │ If not already   │   │   │
└──────────────────┘   │ • Check electrode/paddle   │   │   │
                       │   positions & contact   │   │   │
                       │ • Attempt/Verify: ETT: IV access│   │   │
┌──────────────────┐   │ • Give epinephrine every 3 min │   │ Up to 3 min │
│   CPR   │   │ • Correct reversible causes   │   │   CPR   │
│   1 min   │   │ • Consider buffers   │   │   │
└──────────────────┘   │   antiarrhythmics   │   │   │
                       │   atropine / pacing │   │   │
                       └─────────────────────────────────┘   └──────────────┘

┌───┐
│ Potentially reversible causes: │
│ Hypoxia   │
│ Hypovolaemia   │
│ Hyper/hypokalaemia & metabolic disorders   │
│ Hypothermia   │
│ Tension pneumothorax   │
│ Tamponade   │
│ Toxic/therapeutic disturbances   │
│ Thromboembolic/mechanical obstruction   │
└───┘

The ALS Algorithm for the management of Cardiac Arrest in Adults.
Note that each successive step is based on the assumption that the one before has been unsuccessful.

Fig. 15 Adult Advanced Life Support (1997 Resuscitation Council (UK) Guidelines for use in the United Kingdom).

Resuscitation (6)

Potentially reversible conditions

Paddle position

When the defibrillator is first turned on, check if it is reading the rhythm through the paddles or through the ECG leads. If it is set to the ECG leads, and these have not been attached, then a straight line appears on the monitor screen. This is not asystole, which is an undulating line (Fig. 14, see p. 12). The defibrillator should be switched to read through the paddles. This is the fastest way of determining the rhythm and the need for defibrillation.

The standard paddle positions (Fig. 16) are just to the right of the sternum, below the clavicle, and just outside the position of the normal cardiac apex. However, in refractory ventricular fibrillation, it may be necessary to defibrillate in the anteroposterior direction with the patient on their side. Alternatively, it may be necessary to change the paddles or the defibrillator in case the machine or paddles are faulty.

Tension pneumothorax

This is diagnosed by inserting a hypodermic needle through the second intercostal space in the mid-clavicular line. If the needle is attached to a syringe full of saline, escaping air is detected easily on aspiration (Fig. 17). The needle can be replaced by a large bore cannula, allowing time for the insertion of a chest drain.

Cardiac tamponade

A tamponade is diagnosed and treated by aspiration. A long wide bore needle is inserted just to the left of the xiphoid cartilage, and aimed upwards and backwards towards the left shoulder at 45° to the skin (Fig. 18). An ECG monitor lead attached to the needle shows an altered pattern of electrical activity on the ECG monitor whenever the needle touches the epicardium. The aspiration of even small volumes of blood can considerably increase the cardiac output.

Fig. 16 The correct position for defibrillator paddles.

Fig. 17 Bubbles in the syringe confirming the diagnosis of a pneumothorax.

Fig. 18 Tapping a cardiac tamponade.

Resuscitation (7)

Resuscitation problems

Cardiac massage

If external cardiac massage is not carried out as described in the Resuscitation Council (UK) Guidelines, or if carried out with excessive force, there is a risk of fracturing the patient's ribs (Fig. 19). There are cases described where the atria of the heart have been ruptured. In cases of prolonged resuscitation, the operators should change before fatigue develops, lest the technique varies and results in inefficient resuscitation.

Defibrillator burns

The defibrillator paddles must never make direct contact with the skin, as this will result in burning due to the high skin resistance (Fig. 20). The paddles should never make contact with the ECG leads on the chest wall. Always ensure that fresh gel pads or an appropriate contact gel is used.

Cardiac pacemaker

Be alerted by the presence of a scar and a bulge over the left breast area (Fig. 21). This may indicate that the patient has a cardiac pacemaker in place. If defibrillation is indicated, this can be carried out, but the apical paddle should be kept at least 12.5 cm away from the pacemaker. The pacemaker should not be damaged by the defibrillation, but there is a risk that current will be conducted down the pacemaker electrode, and this can result in a burn where the tip lies against the myocardium. This could subsequently alter the pacing threshold.

Fig. 19 Bruising and fractured ribs at post mortem after prolonged resuscitation.

Fig. 20 Defibrillator burns resulting from poor technique.

Fig. 21 A patient with a cardiac pacemaker implant.

Resuscitation (8)

Central venous cannulation

This procedure is normally elective and it is not a method of choice for emergency resuscitation, where direct cannulation of forearm or antecubital veins is quicker and easier. Short wide bore cannulas give much higher flow rates. In experienced hands, these techniques can be used to give resuscitation drugs or for the passing of a temporary pacing wire.

Internal jugular vein cannulation

The patient is placed in a 15° head down position to distend the neck veins and minimize the risk of air embolism. The head is turned to the opposite side and the skin is thoroughly cleaned. With the appropriate needle and catheter, locate the apex of the triangle formed by the sternal and clavicular heads or the sternomastoid muscle. Advance the needle through the skin at an angle of approximately 30° to the horizontal and aim for the ipsilateral nipple. Successful puncture is made at the depth of between 2 and 5 cm (Fig. 22).

Supraclavicular approach to the subclavian vein

With the patient in the above position and with the skin cleansed, the anatomical landmark is the lateral edge of the clavicular head of the sternomastoid, where it meets the clavicle. Place a finger in the angle between the clavicle and the lateral edge of the clavicular head of the sternomastoid and at a point 1 cm behind the clavicle, insert the needle, hold it horizontal and advance it towards a point midway between the sternal notch and the manubriosternal joint (Fig. 23). Blood should be aspirated at 2–3 cm depth.

Infraclavicular approach to the subclavian

With the patient in the position described above, insert the needle and cannula just below the junction of the medial one-third and lateral two-thirds of the clavicle. The needle is held horizontal and advanced towards the upper aspect of the sternoclavicular joint on that side (Fig. 24). Blood should be aspirated at approximately 3–5 cm depth.

All of the above procedures carry potentially serious risks, the most common being a pneumothorax.

Fig. 22 Approach to the internal jugular vein.

Fig. 23 Supraclavicular approach to the subclavian vein.

Fig. 24 Infraclavicular approach to the subclavian vein.

3 / Head injuries

Head injuries are common and often present to an A & E department following a road traffic accident or a fight. In these situations, alcohol may play a large part in the patient's clinical state. The smell of alcohol is no indication of the volume which might have been consumed. Alcohol may confuse the issue because there are common features between alcohol excess and a head injury such as loss of consciousness, confusion and aggression. Always assume that these are the result of the head injury rather than alcohol. If in doubt, admit the patient for observation.

Level of consciousness

Loss of consciousness following trauma may result from a head injury or hypovolaemia and hypoxia. These must be corrected and the patient's neurological state reassessed, as well as treating other concurrent injuries.

Scalp wounds

These are initially difficult to assess (Fig. 25) due to blood in the hair. When the wound has been cleaned, it may look less severe than was originally thought (Fig. 26). Feel gently with a gloved finger in the wound to detect any underlying fracture (Fig. 27). Scalp wounds may bleed heavily but they are not a cause of hypovolaemia in adults—if present, look for another cause.

Fig. 25 Scalp laceration on arrival.

Fig. 26 Scalp laceration after cleaning.

Fig. 27 Depressed skull fracture.

Skull fractures

An increase of the intracranial pressure may cause compression of the oculomotor nerve against the tentorium cerebelli and produce ipsilateral dilatation of the pupil. It is important to exclude other causes of unequal pupils such as direct trauma to the eye, the application of medication (Fig. 28) or a glass eye.

Anterior cranial fossa fractures can cause cerebrospinal fluid (CSF) rhinorrhoea, marked periorbital haematomata (panda eyes), associated with subconjunctival haemorrhage (Fig. 29). Bloody CSF rhinorrhoea may be identified by dropping some of the fluid on to blotting paper—if CSF is present, there will be a central ring of blood with a peripheral halo of CSF.

Middle cranial fossa fractures produce a haemotympanum and, if the membrane is ruptured, blood and CSF leakage from the ear (Fig. 30). Posterior auricular bruising may also occur (Battle's sign)—usually later.

It is more important to observe the patient's level of consciousness than to take X-rays of the skull. Skull X-rays are notoriously difficult to interpret, particularly if the patient is restless and the quality of the film is suboptimal. Computerized tomography is the examination of choice to diagnose intracranial haemorrhage.

Fig. 28 Unequal pupils—dilated with cyclopentolate.

Fig. 29 Panda eyes.

Fig. 30 Blood from ear.

Trauma

Aetiology

A direct blow to the eye may damage the eyelids, globe or bony wall of the orbit and, of these, the floor is the most often injured.

Clinical features

Fracture. A fracture produces a periorbital haematoma, local tenderness, a palpable step and a subconjunctival haemorrhage. If the posterior limit of the haemorrhage is not visible, assume that there is a fracture. There may be altered sensation in the distribution of the infraorbital nerve. A fracture which involves the floor of the orbit but not the free margin is a blow-out fracture. This, in addition to the features described above, produces enophthalmos and trapping of the infraorbital structures (Fig. 31). X-rays confirm the fracture and there is opacity of the maxillary sinus (Fig. 32). Tomography or a CT scan may be required to delineate the blow-out fracture.

Hyphaema. A hyphaema is a collection of blood in the anterior chamber, resulting from damage to vessels on the iris (Fig. 33).

Treatment

The patient is advised not to blow their nose and prophylactic antibiotics are usually prescribed. Displaced zygomatic fractures require surgical correction as do those blow-out fractures which trap the infraorbital structures.

A patient suffering from a hyphaema should be referred to an ophthalmologist. If the patient does not rest, there is a risk of further bleeding and this is associated with a rise of the intraocular pressure which may require specific treatment.

Fig. 31 Limitation of upward gaze resulting from a blow-out fracture.

Fig. 32 'Tear drop' soft tissue swelling at the roof of the maxillary antrum.

Fig. 33 A hyphaema.

Pain

Aetiology

Pain may result from surface structures or deeper structures. Surface pain results from conjunctival or scleral irritation. This may be due to a foreign body, primary conjunctivitis (Fig. 34), a corneal abrasion, scleritis or episcleritis.

Clinical features

The visual acuity should be assessed in both eyes using normal visual aids. It is usually normal. There may be photophobia, epiphora, conjunctival redness and blepharospasm. The whole of the anterior surface of the globe must be examined carefully and the eyelids everted (Fig. 35). Given a history of a high velocity fragment, X-rays must be taken of the orbital contents to exclude an intraocular foreign body even if one is seen on the surface. Staining of the cornea with fluorescein shows any corneal epithelial defect.

Treatment

Metallic corneal foreign bodies. When seen within the first few hours, these may be removed easily under local anaesthesia but, if present for longer, there may be an associated 'rust-ring' (Fig. 36). This is difficult to remove in its entirety and it is preferable to apply a firm eye-pad, give a topical antibiotic and refer to an ophthalmologist at 72 h for its removal.

Conjunctivitis. This condition is treated with topical antibiotics for 72 h and a firm eye-pad.

Scleritis and episcleritis. These are occasionally associated with systemic disorders such as rheumatoid disease and inflammatory bowel disease, and the eye condition is best treated by an ophthalmologist.

Fig. 34 Bacterial conjunctivitis.

Fig. 35 Metallic foreign body beneath the upper eyelid.

Fig. 36 Rust-ring at 48 h after removal of a foreign body.

Other important causes of pain

These include the following:
- a dendritic ulcer
- acute glaucoma
- acute iritis
- perforating injury.

Clinical features

Dendritic ulcer: a corneal ulcer of viral aetiology. It causes symptoms of conjunctivitis but does not respond to antibiotics. Fluorescein staining reveals the typical branched ulcer (Fig. 37). Topical steroids are absolutely contraindicated.

Acute glaucoma: a condition associated with pain in the eye and diminished visual acuity. The globe is palpably firm, the cornea hazy and the pupil oval and non-reactive to light. It may arise de novo or be secondary to anticholinergic drugs.

Iritis: inflammation of the anterior uveal tract which causes intense pain and photophobia. The pupil is small and the redness is initially around the cornea (Fig. 38). The consensual light reflex causes pain in the affected eye.

Perforating injury: should be suspected with a history of a high velocity missile, e.g. metal striking metal. There may be a scleral or corneal wound which may not be obvious. The iris may prolapse through a corneal wound producing a tear-shaped pupil (Fig. 39).

Treatment

Early referral to an ophthalmologist should be made in all of these cases since serious complications can develop or the systemic disease which precipitated the condition requires investigation and treatment.

Fig. 37 Fluorescein-stained dendritic ulcer under ultraviolet light.

Fig. 38 Acute iritis.

Fig. 39 Iris prolapse through a corneal wound.

Dental problems

Trauma

Subluxation or dislocation of a tooth results from trauma. If a tooth has been dislocated, it can be stored in milk or in the buccal sulcus pending relocation.

Treatment

The tooth should be cleaned carefully and replaced in its socket as soon as possible, then splinted. The longer the delay in reducing a subluxed or dislocated tooth, the greater the chance of damage to the neurovascular structures in the pulp (Fig. 40). If a tooth has been dislocated and cannot be found, X-ray the chest to ensure that it has not been inhaled. The usual site at which it will lodge is in the right main bronchus (Fig. 41).

Treatment

The bleeding socket

This is treated by rolling a gauze swab and placing it directly across the socket. The patient is advised to bite firmly for 15 min. If unsuccessful (Fig. 42), a horizontal mattress suture may be placed across the neck of the socket. It does not close the socket but tightens the gingiva, so arresting mucosal bleeding. If this fails, a plug of a haemostatic material should be inserted into the socket prior to suture.

Fig. 40 Discoloration of a dislocated tooth resulting from damage to the pulp.

Fig. 41 Inhaled tooth in the right main bronchus.

Fig. 42 A bleeding tooth socket.

Nasal problems

Trauma
This may result in deformity and marked swelling.

Treatment

There is no need to X-ray the nose unless a compound fracture is suspected. The nasal bridge is tender and deviated (Fig. 43) and this is best seen from above. The patency of the nasal airways should be checked and a septal haematoma (Fig. 44) looked for. This looks like a cherry in the middle of the nose and, if present, immediate ENT referral should be made since the septal cartilage may be rendered ischaemic and will perforate, particularly if an abscess develops. A patient with a suspected nasal fracture is usually referred to an ENT surgeon between 5 and 10 days from the date of injury to decide if reduction is necessary.

Epistaxis
This occurs usually at the extremes of life and may result from trauma, mucosal inflammation or spontaneous haemorrhage (Fig. 45) from atherosclerotic vessels associated occasionally with hypertension. The septum may bleed anteriorly from Little's area or from more posteriorly.

Treatment

- *Anterior bleeding* may be controlled readily by pinching the nose firmly, but occasionally it is necessary to cauterize the vessel or pack the nose.
- *Posterior bleeding* should be treated by an ENT surgeon since this usually requires packing and may necessitate early surgery.

Fig. 43 Septal haematoma.

Fig. 44 Frontal view of a deviated nasal bridge.

Fig. 45 Hereditary haemorrhagic telangiectasia resulting in epistaxis.

Lip injuries

Full thickness wounds are common and are due to direct trauma from outside, or a tooth biting through the lip.

Treatment The wound edges should be débrided and then closed in layers to avoid the development of a salivary fistula. A wound through the vermilion border (Fig. 46) must be repaired very carefully since the slightest irregularity of the scar leaves a cosmetically obvious appearance.

Mucosal lacerations heal very well. They initially become macerated and ulcerated and the patient should be advised to use a saline or antiseptic mouthwash and take care with dental hygiene.

Jaw injuries

Dislocation

Dislocation usually occurs without trauma. Typically, the patient yawns, feels pain in front of the ear and is unable to close the mouth properly (Fig. 47).

Treatment X-rays confirm the dislocation and reduction is effected easily by firm downward and backward pressure on the lower molar teeth.

Fracture

A fracture of the mandible is not always obvious clinically. Palpate carefully the whole of the mandible and look for misalignment of the teeth, swelling, bleeding or sublingual bruising which, if present, is pathognomonic of the diagnosis until proven otherwise. X-ray the mandible and be careful to maintain the patient's airway, particularly if the level of consciousness is depressed.

Fig. 46 Wound at the vermilion border.

Fig. 47 Unilateral dislocation resulting in deviation of the chin.

Throat problems

Clinical features

Patients often present complaining of having swallowed something which has lodged in the throat. The position of the foreign body is not well localized and there is dysphagia. Rarely there may be dyspnoea and dysphonia and, if the foreign body has perforated the airway, there will be surgical emphysema.

Examination

Inspect the mouth carefully, the tonsillar area (Fig. 48) and the posterior third of the tongue, behind the vallate papillae. It is possible to examine the larynx indirectly with a mirror, but this takes practice and the patient's confidence must be gained. X-rays of the soft tissues of the neck may visualize a foreign body (Fig. 49) and show any associated surgical emphysema. However, foreign bodies are often difficult to identify, particularly in a patient with heavily calcified laryngeal cartilages.

Treatment

If the foreign body is identified in the oropharynx, remove it. It may be necessary to spray the oropharynx with topical local anaesthetic and, if this is done, warn the patient not to eat or drink until sensation has returned to normal. When the foreign body has been removed, warn the patient to expect the abnormal sensation to persist for several days until the mucosal wound has healed.

If the foreign body is not visible and the patient has significant symptoms such as drooling of saliva, dysphagia or dyspnoea, ask for an urgent ENT opinion.

Fig. 48 Fish bone lodged in the right tonsillar area.

Fig. 49 Glass foreign body in the oesophagus at the C7/T1 level.

Inflammatory conditions

Aetiology

Otitis externa: occurs commonly in those engaged in water sports. The inflammation may be allergic, bacterial or fungal in origin (Fig. 50).

Otitis media: occurs most commonly in children as part of an upper respiratory tract infection.

Clinical features

Otitis externa: causes itching of the external ear canal, a watery discharge and conductive deafness.

Otitis media: causes severe throbbing pain, fever and conductive deafness.

Examination

There is tenderness of the tragus and movements of the jaw are painful. There may be excoriation of the skin and the external ear canal is oedematous.
  Otitis media is associated with redness and bulging of the eardrum.

Treatment

Otitis externa: local cleansing along with instillation of combined steroid and antibiotic drops or cream. Alternatively, a wick soaked in this preparation may be inserted and changed after 24 h. The condition may be slow to resolve.

Otitis media: systemic antibiotics. If treated inadequately, otitis media with an effusion may develop in children. If there is frank pus behind the eardrum, it should be drained surgically by an ENT surgeon.

Fig. 50 Otitis externa.

Non-infective conditions

Aetiology

- A perichondral haematoma (Fig. 51) is caused by direct trauma to the external ear.
- Wounds through the cartilage of the ear are traumatic in origin (Fig. 53).
- Traumatic perforation of the eardrum is due to a direct injury, e.g. scratching the ear canal with a pointed object, or by a high pressure air wave as a result of a blow to the side of the head.
- Foreign bodies may be in the meatus or embedded in the pinna (Fig. 52).

Clinical features

The perichondrium is stripped away from the cartilage and there is a boggy, tender swelling.

Perforation of the eardrum leads to conductive deafness and a bloody discharge.

Treatment

The haematoma should be aspirated under sterile conditions and a firm dressing applied to the contours of the ear. Alternatively, a small suction drain may be introduced via the posterior surface of the ear to drain the haematoma and minimize the chance of its recurrence. This is an ENT procedure.

When an extensive injury damages skin and cartilage, the cartilaginous skeleton should be reconstructed carefully. The irregular skin edges should be trimmed to allow accurate closure to obtain a cosmetically acceptable result.

Meatal foreign bodies are often small round objects and are best removed under general anaesthetic, but those in the pinna can usually be removed under local anaesthetic from the back of the pinna.

Fig. 51 A perichondral haematoma.

Fig. 52 Following nickel allergy, the ear stud has become embedded in the pinna.

Fig. 53 A sutured machete wound to the ear.

Pain

Aetiology

Sprain. A sprain of the cervical spine occurs most commonly in a rear impact road traffic accident. It causes hyperextension of the cervical spine followed rapidly by flexion (whiplash injury).

Torticollis. Spontaneous onset of pain in the neck may be due to acute torticollis (Fig. 54). This is due to spasm in the large muscles of the neck. It is of unknown aetiology.

Clinical features

Sprain. There may be transient neurological symptoms and the neck is usually pain free initially. Pain and stiffness develop gradually and X-rays show a straight cervical spine which is evidence of spasm.

Torticollis. This occurs in young adults and is associated with the neck held flexed and the head rotated to one side. There are no abnormal neurological signs.

Treatment

Sprain. There are several methods which include immobilization in a firm or soft cervical collar (Figs 55 & 56) until the patient is pain free. There is a trend towards early mobilization with or without active physiotherapy. The acute symptoms of a whiplash injury may last up to 8 weeks but a less intense discomfort may develop and this may last for months.

Torticollis. This resolves quickly and medication with painkillers and muscle relaxants (such as diazepam) resolve the symptoms within a few days.

Fig. 54 Torticollis.

Fig. 55 Anterior view of a soft cervical collar.

Fig. 56 Posterior view of a soft cervical collar showing the Velcro fastener.

Wounds

Aetiology

They may be self-inflicted (Fig. 57) or due to an assault (Fig. 58). In either case, the motive is death. Occasionally a wound may result from an accident.

Clinical features

The self-inflicted wound usually has 'intention' marks. These are short, superficial wounds which increase in depth and length until the major wound is produced. Wounds resulting from an assault are usually single and deep.

Treatment

Cover with a moist dressing and apply direct pressure. The patient can sit up and this will decrease haemorrhage; however, this position increases the risk of air embolism. If the patient is hypotensive, or there are other injuries present, it may be necessary to lie them down, but this will tend to increase the haemorrhage. Other injuries must be sought and treated. Clamping vessels blindly must not be attempted.

Wounds which penetrate the platysma should be explored formally in theatre but more superficial wounds may be sutured in the department after careful inspection.

Damage to the upper airway should be assessed carefully and an experienced anaesthetist and ENT surgeon consulted early.

Fig. 57 Self-inflicted throat laceration.

Fig. 58 Gunshot wound to the neck.

Non-penetrating injuries

Aetiology

- *Direct injuries* occur most commonly as a result of a fall, sport or an assault.
- *Indirect injuries* occur in pathologically weakened bone such as in postmenopausal women, patients on steroids or those with disseminated malignancy.

Clinical features

There is marked tenderness over the area of the injury. A deceleration injury resulting from a road traffic accident produces characteristic bruising (Fig. 59) and an ECG may show evidence of myocardial injury.

The diagnosis of a rib fracture does not require an X-ray, but an X-ray is required if there is suspicion of associated pathology such as a chest infection or a pneumothorax.

Treatment

Strapping the ribs around half the circumference of the chest wall (Fig. 60) gives good pain relief and does not limit respiration, provided that an elasticated strapping is used. Analgesia must be provided and this may be systemic or by a regional nerve block. Advice regarding breathing exercises should be given to minimize the likelihood of a chest infection developing.

Penetrating injuries

These are uncommon and are due to assault (Fig. 61) or accident. The major life-threatening conditions of a tension pneumothorax or cardiac tamponade must be sought and treated immediately. Penetrating cardiac injuries must be treated by immediate thoracotomy and closure of the myocardial defect.

Fig. 59 Seat belt marks across the chest and abdomen.

Fig. 60 Rib strapping.

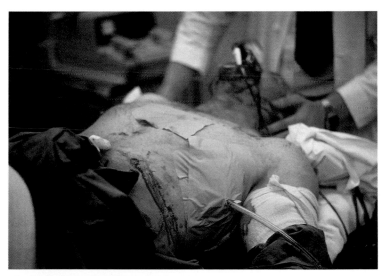

Fig. 61 Stabbing to the chest and abdomen.

9 / The shoulder

Stability of the glenohumeral joint is sacrificed in favour of the large range of movement which is permitted. The bony contours and labrum glenoidale contribute little to stability, this being afforded primarily by the tendons of the rotator cuff and the ligaments.

Anterior dislocation

This occurs typically in young adults and results from a fall on to the outstretched hand.

Clinical features

There is pain, spasm and the rounded contour of the deltoid is replaced by the square contour of the acromion (Fig. 62). Neuropraxia of the brachial plexus or axillary nerve occurs infrequently but should be sought prior to reduction.

Treatment

There are several methods of reduction, including the Hippocratic, Kocher, Stimson and Milch manoeuvres. The technique used should be dictated by local policy. Entonox may suffice as the method of analgesia but an opiate is usually required in addition. General or regional anaesthesia may be needed in more muscular patients.

Posterior dislocation

This occurs much less frequently and is seen particularly in epileptics or those having suffered an electric shock.

Clinical features

The contour of the shoulder is normal. The X-ray reveals the 'light-bulb' deformity (symmetry of the humeral head) and it stands off more than usual from the glenoid (Fig. 63). An axial view is essential to confirm the diagnosis (Fig. 64).

Fig. 62 Anterior dislocation of the left shoulder.

Fig. 63 Anterior X-ray of a posterior dislocation of the left shoulder.

Fig. 64 Axial X-ray of a posterior dislocation of the left shoulder.

Painful arc

This is pain arising from the shoulder itself or the associated soft tissues and is felt typically in the middle one-third of abduction (Fig. 65).

Aetiology

- Calcific bursitis (Fig. 66)
- Degenerative rotator cuff disease
- Degenerative disease of the acromioclavicular joint

Clinical features

The pain may be of spontaneous onset, radiates to the insertion of the deltoid muscle and is of an aching nature. There may be limitation of rotation at the shoulder joint.

Treatment

This is directed at reducing local inflammation using physiotherapy, non-steroidal anti-inflammatory agents and maintaining mobility by gentle exercises. Local steroid injections may be of benefit but strict asepsis must be observed.

Acromioclavicular injuries

Acromioclavicular separation may be divided into 1st, 2nd and 3rd degree, depending upon the amount of separation seen radiographically.

Aetiology

A fall on to the point of the shoulder, usually in young sportsmen.

Clinical features

Local tenderness and deformity (Fig. 67). There is painful limitation of movement and X-rays exclude a fracture of the outer end of the clavicle.

Treatment

Analgesia and a triangular bandage followed by gentle exercises produce good results, although the deformity generally persists.

Fig. 65 Painful limitation of abduction.

Fig. 66 Calcification in the subacromial bursa.

Fig. 67 Complete separation of the left acromioclavicular joint.

Damage to the biceps muscle

Aetiology

The long head of the biceps muscle is thought to rupture due to avascular degeneration and thus is a condition of the over 50s. The distal attachment may rupture due to similar pathology or due to scarring from previous injury. A direct blow to the biceps may result from an assault or contact sport and cause an intramuscular haematoma.

Clinical features

The patient will generally have been stressing his arm when he feels something go. If the injury has occurred recently, there will be pain on contracting the biceps. The free head contracts up or down the arm and appears as a swelling over its anterior aspect (Fig. 68). After a few days, heavy bruising may develop down the arm (Fig. 69).

Treatment

Rupture of the long head is treated conservatively using analgesia, a broad arm sling and then mobilization. Distal rupture is usually treated operatively because of the weakness of elbow flexion produced by damage to the tendon.

Direct damage to the biceps muscle may result in myositis ossificans and subsequent fibrosis within the muscle belly (Fig. 70). Such scarring is likely to be stimulated by early, vigorous mobilization so this must be avoided.

Fig. 68 Rupture of the long head of the biceps

Fig. 69 Heavy bruising resulting from an acute rupture of the biceps tendon.

Fig. 70 Scarring of the muscle belly resulting from a previous direct injury.

Trauma

Aetiology

The usual mechanism is a fall on to the outstretched hand although direct trauma may also result in bony or ligamentous damage.

Clinical features

There may be swelling and deformity at the elbow (Fig. 71). The olecranon and epicondyles normally form an equilateral triangle—dislocation disrupts this relationship whilst a supracondylar fracture maintains it. A fracture of the olecranon produces marked local swelling, bruising and the bony prominence may not be palpable. There may be abnormal movement with crepitus around the joint and it is particularly important to check the distal neurovascular function since urgent reduction must be effected if there is any compromise.

X-ray

This demonstrates the bony injury but care must be taken in children to check the epiphyseal centres (Fig. 72) which can be displaced minimally but cause significant functional deficit subsequently. If there is no obvious bone or joint injury, check for the presence of an effusion. This raises the intracapsular but extrasynovial fat pads which appear as dark sail-like shadows anterior and posterior to the distal humerus (Fig. 73).

Treatment

A displaced injury must be reduced urgently. Displaced epicondylar or olecranon fractures are fixed internally whilst displaced radial head fractures are either excised or fixed, according to local policy. Non-displaced fractures of the radial head are treated conservatively.

Fig. 71 Posterior dislocation of the elbow.

Fig. 72 Separation of the medial epicondylar epiphysis.

Fig. 73 Anterior and posterior fat pads.

Tendinitis

Aetiology

Epicondylitis and biceps tendinitis are due to unaccustomed repetitive activity. Epicondylitis is rarely due to playing tennis or golf.

Clinical features

There is pain and tenderness over the tendon attachment. Resisted movements of the wrist produce pain at the elbow in the case of epicondylitis (Fig. 74). Biceps tendinitis is associated with pain caused by resisted flexion of the elbow (Fig. 75) or resisted supination of the forearm.

Treatment

The elbow should be rested and a course of non-steroidal anti-inflammatory drugs should be given. If the symptoms fail to resolve, an injection of steroid and local anaesthetic around the point of maximum tenderness will help to relieve the symptoms. It is important to make the injection correctly—injection directly into a tendon is associated with tendon rupture and injection into the subcutaneous tissue is associated with skin atrophy. Strict asepsis must be observed and up to three injections may be given at any one site at intervals of at least one month.

Rarely, epicondylitis is resistant to conservative treatment and surgical release of the tendinous aponeurosis is required.

Fig. 74 Lateral epicondylar pain produced by resisted extension of the wrist.

Fig. 75 Biceps tendinitis.

Colles' fracture

A Colles' fracture is produced by a fall on to the outstretched hand and occurs most commonly in elderly women. It results in a dinner-fork deformity of the wrist (Fig. 76).

Treatment

The need for reduction depends upon the position of the bone and the patient's age. Reduction may be under general or regional anaesthesia.

Bier's block. This is a simple technique (Fig. 77) which gives good regional anaesthesia using an appropriate local anaesthetic agent. A full pre-anaesthetic assessment should be made and the patient fasted as for a general anaesthetic. As with any regional anaesthetic technique, full resuscitation equipment must be available.

Swollen hand

Following injury, the hand may become markedly swollen. Resultant immobility of the hand and a dependent posture compound the swelling.

Treatment

The patient must have the limb elevated in a high arm sling and be encouraged to exercise the fingers and thumb at least once each hour.

Median nerve compression

This occurs usually secondarily to trauma or rheumatoid disease. The nerve is trapped in the carpal tunnel and causes pain in the hand and radial $3\frac{1}{2}$ digits with altered sensation in this area. Tinel's sign is positive (Fig. 78), i.e. tapping over the median nerve produces tingling within its distribution.

Treatment

Treatment may be conservative, by elevation of the limb, but surgical decompression may be required.
  Rarely, median nerve compression may be associated with hypothyroidism or fluid retention in pregnancy.

Fig. 76 Dinner-fork deformity of a Colles' fracture.

Fig. 77 Bier's block—note the double cuff.

Fig. 78 Tinel's sign being elicited.

Lunate dislocation

This can dislocate alone or be associated with a fracture of the scaphoid and/or triquetral. The injury is usually missed if not specifically sought.

X-ray signs

- The abnormal spacing between the proximal carpal bones (Fig. 79).
- The triangular appearance of the lunate.
- The loss of the three crescents—the lunate sits in the crescent of the distal radius and the capitate sits in the crescent of the lunate (Fig. 80).

Smith's fracture

This occurs as a result of a fall on to the back of the hand. It is the reverse of a Colles' fracture in that the distal fragment is angulated anteriorly (Fig. 81).

Treatment

Reduction is effected under anaesthesia with traction on the supinated forearm. A full arm cast is applied with the elbow at a right angle, the forearm in supination and the wrist dorsiflexed.

Fracture check-list

With any fracture, *always*:
- ascertain the mechanism of injury
- check whether there could be more than one injury
- examine the joint above and below the site of the injury.

In the forearm, do not forget the Galeazzi and Monteggia fracture–dislocations.

Fig. 79 Anteroposterior view of a perilunar dislocation.

Fig. 80 Lateral view of a perilunar dislocation.

Fig. 81 A Smith's fracture.

Soft tissue conditions

Wrist sprains are common. They generally result from a hyperextension injury and can cause considerable discomfort which will persist for 4–6 weeks. The problem is to exclude a bony injury such as a scaphoid fracture.

Tenosynovitis

This term is readily used by patients, usually in relation to wrist pain secondary to unaccustomed repetitive activity such as home decorating or using a computer keyboard.

Tenosynovitis results from inflammation between the tendon and tendon sheath. The classical site is over the abductor pollicis longus and extensor pollicis brevis tendons on the radial side of the wrist. It may progress to tendon sheath stenosis: de Quervain's disease.

Clinical features

There is swelling over the tendon (Fig. 82) and crepitation over the tendon sheath when the thumb is moved. Finkelstein's test (Fig. 83) involves the patient placing the thumb in the palm of the hand and gripping it by the fingers. Ulnar deviation of the hand produces pain.

Treatment

Rest is very important and may be enforced by immobilization in a cast. If unsuccessful, a local steroid injection into the tendon sheath will help. Stenosis of the sheath requires surgical release.

Fig. 82 Swelling over the tendons on the radial side of the wrist.

Fig. 83 Finkelstein's test.

The fractured scaphoid

Aetiology

This is due to a hyperextension injury, typically by falling on to the outstretched hand. It may occur in any age group but is most likely in young adult males.

Clinical features

There is tenderness in the anatomical snuffbox (Fig. 84), but it is important to palpate and compare tenderness in the right and left anatomical snuff boxes. Also palpate the dorsal and ventral aspects of the scaphoid to elicit tenderness (Fig. 85) and assess pain produced by axial compression of the thumb metacarpal on to the trapezium and thence the scaphoid (Fig. 86).

X-rays

These should be anteroposterior, lateral and the two 45° obliques. If a fracture is apparent radiologically, or any of the above diagnostic criteria are met, a forearm cast should be applied which immobilizes the thumb metacarpophalangeal joint. If a fracture is not confirmed, the cast should be removed at about 10 days and a further set of radiographs taken. Persisting tenderness and a normal second set of X-rays should be treated by further cast immobilization and a bone scan requested. This may give a definitive answer but care should be exercised in patients who exhibit arthritic changes at the base of the thumb since this can give a false positive result.

Fig. 84 Tenderness in the anatomical snuff box.

Fig. 85 Palpation of the dorsal and ventral surfaces of the scaphoid.

Fig. 86 Axial compression of the thumb.

Tendon injuries

Aetiology

A closed injury of the extensor tendon in the finger disrupts the attachment of the extensor tendon to the middle or distal phalanx, causing a boutonnière or mallet deformity respectively. A hyperextension injury may avulse one of the flexor tendons or the volar plate at the base of the middle phalanx.

Clinical features

Mallet finger (Fig. 87).   This is associated with loss of active extension of the distal interphalangeal joint. X-rays may show an avulsed fragment of bone.

Boutonnière deformity (Fig. 88).   This is due to the head of the middle phalanx prolapsing dorsally between the two slips of the extensor tendon and through the extensor hood, producing the characteristic deformity.

Volar plate injuries.   Injury to the volar plate produces fusiform swelling, local pain and limitation of movement at the proximal interphalangeal joint.

Open injuries.   These do not necessarily produce a characteristic posture or loss of function.

Treatment

- A boutonnière or mallet finger is treated conservatively by splinting for 6 weeks (Fig. 89).
- Volar plate injuries are treated conservatively by neighbour strapping for up to 2 weeks followed by active mobilization.
- Open injuries to the tendons must be suspected when presented with any wound on the wrist or hand. It is important to assess the function of all deep structures. If there is any doubt, referral to a hand surgeon must be made.

Fig. 87 A mallet deformity.

Fig. 88 A boutonnière deformity.

Fig. 89 A Capener and mallet splint.

Nail injuries

Aetiology

The major cause of injury to the nail and distal phalanx is a crush injury. Less commonly, direct wounds are responsible.

Clinical features

A subungual haematoma (Fig. 90) may be associated with a fracture of the distal phalanx. It is exquisitely tender and X-rays reveal any associated fracture.

Dislocation of the nail root from beneath the cuticle (Fig. 91) may also be associated with a fracture of the distal phalanx. The fracture is typically transverse with anterior angulation of the distal fragment.

Treatment

Subungual haematoma. The haematoma is drained by a small hole drilled through the nail. The hole may be made with a red-hot paper clip, a sterile hypodermic needle or a commercially available drill. Early evacuation of liquid blood is much more effective in relieving pain than attempted later evacuation of semi-clotted blood. If there is a fracture, antibiotics should be given.

Dislocated nail. The nail should be replaced carefully (Fig. 92) for two reasons: firstly to act as a splint for the distal bony fragment and to hold the distal soft tissues in place; and secondly, to prevent damage to the developing nail caused by adhesions between the cuticle and germinal part of the nail bed (Fig. 93).

Fig. 90 A subungual haematoma.

Fig. 91 Dislocation of the nail root.

Fig. 92 Reduced nail root, supported by a horizontal mattress suture.

Fig. 93 Ridging of the nail resulting from damage to the germinal epithelium.

Fingertip injuries

Aetiology

Full thickness skin loss from the tip of the finger or thumb may be caused by either a sharp or blunt injury.

Treatment

Incomplete amputation. The fingertip may be reconstructed carefully using either steristrips or lightly placed sutures and has a good chance of survival, particularly in children.

Complete amputation (Fig. 94). This requires tissue cover. If bone is proud of the soft tissue, the patient should be referred for definitive surgery but, if the bone is not proud, it can be managed in the A & E department. Replantation may be considered, particularly if the amputation has been caused by a clean, incised injury rather than a tearing, crush injury. It is most likely to be attempted in one of the radial three digits because of their importance to the grip.

Surgical cover by means of a skin graft may be used but this often creates a fingertip with markedly impaired sensation, an obviously deformed fingertip (Fig. 95) and an obvious, initially very painful, graft donor site (Fig. 96) which leaves a permanent scar.

Conservative treatment, using silver sulphadiazine cream or a non-adherent tulle-gras dressing, allows spontaneous healing within 4–6 weeks. This produces a cosmetically good result, the sensation of the tip returns to near normal, and it avoids the scar of a graft donor site.

Fig. 94 Complete amputation of the fingertip.

Fig. 95 Previously amputated fingertip treated by grafting. Note the nail spike.

Fig. 96 Graft donor site from same source as Figure 95.

Infections

Aetiology

These may develop as a primary infection but more commonly occur secondary to a trivial wound or retained foreign body. The infecting organisms include streptococci and staphylococci, but a wide variety of other organisms may be seen, particularly in butchers or gardeners.

Clinical features

There is marked swelling resulting from the inflammatory oedema occurring in an area where the tissue is very lax. Pyogenic infection may produce a collection of pus in one of the deep palmar spaces (Fig. 97) and there may be lymphangitis and systemic upset.

Following a relatively minor injury, there may be the sinister complication of flexor tendon sheath infection associated with tissue necrosis (Fig. 98). This is characterized by exquisitely painful active or passive movement of the affected finger, with tenderness along the flexor tendon proximal to the site of obvious infection.

Treatment

This involves elevation of the limb, high dose antibiotics and frequent review.

If there is systemic upset or clinical evidence of any pus collection in a palmar space or tendon sheath, urgent decompression must be undertaken to prevent damage to the palmar structures or fibrous adhesions to the tendon.

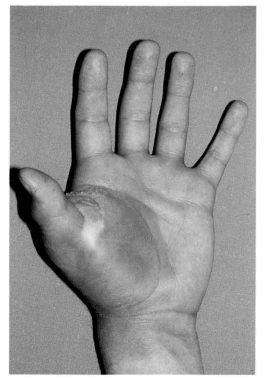

Fig. 97 Pyogenic infection in the hand.

Fig. 98 Skin infection and necrosis resulting from deep-seated infection.

Miscellaneous problems

Degloving injuries

These result from catching the hand in machinery or catching a ring on something (Fig. 99). The ring cuts into the soft tissue at the base of the finger and tears it distally. There is impairment of the neurovascular function and the underlying tendon or bone may be damaged. Early referral to a hand unit is indicated since microsurgery might be contemplated if the degree of nerve and vessel damage is not too great.

Fractures

Non-displaced fractures of the fingers or hand are usually treated conservatively by neighbour strapping or resting in a cast. However, even with apparently 'non-displaced' fractures, it is important to check that there has been no rotation of the metacarpal or phalanx and, if present, this should be corrected prior to immobilization. If this is not undertaken there may be significant functional disability caused by overlapping of the digits when the patient makes a fist (Fig. 101).

High pressure injection

High pressure oil, paint or air injection into a digit is an apparently innocuous injury (Fig. 100) but must be treated urgently. The foreign material passes for a surprisingly great distance into the digit and requires early surgical evacuation of the foreign material and débridement of damaged tissue. The injected oil or paint is very irritant to the tissues and may also result in impairment of the circulation.

Fig. 99 Ring injury to a finger.

Fig. 100 Innocent-looking high pressure injection wound from brake fluid.

Fig. 101 Rotation of the little finger secondary to a spiral fracture.

Aetiology

- *Haemorrhoids* are dilated veins of a plexus at and below the anorectal ring. They are of unknown aetiology but are more common in postpartum females.
- *Perianal haematoma*, usually occurring spontaneously.
- *Fissure-in-ano*, a tear in the anal mucosa which results in painful spasm of the anal sphincter.
- *Threadworm infection* in children.

Symptoms

These include pain, pruritus and spotting of blood on the underwear. Haemorrhoids may enlarge and be extruded through the anus and may be classified as first, second or third degree, depending on the propensity with which they prolapse and the ease with which they can be reduced (Fig. 102). A perianal haematoma causes a localized, tender swelling at the anal margin. Threadworms cause irritation at night when they lay their eggs in the perianal region.

Treatment

Third degree (irreducible) haemorrhoids   cause considerable local pain and may bleed, ulcerate or thrombose. This is a surgical emergency and should be treated either by reduction or excision under general anaesthesia.

Perianal haematoma: relieved instantly by incision and evacuation.

Fissure-in-ano: treatment usually involves stretching of the anal sphincter under general anaesthesia, or a lateral anal sphincterotomy.

Threadworms (Fig. 103):   respond to oral medication, such as piperazine or mebendazole.

Fig. 102 Third degree haemorrhoids.

Fig. 103 Threadworm on a specimen of faeces.

Infective conditions

Aetiology

- This is usually secondary to infection of a hair follicle or secondary to trauma to the mucosa of the anal canal (Fig. 104).
- A pilonidal sinus is one which is related to an area of skin which has been irritated by hair. Typically, it occurs over the lower sacrum or coccyx (Fig. 105), but may also occur on the hand, such as that of a hairdresser.

Symptoms

Pain is of a deep, throbbing nature and increases when sitting or straining to evacuate the bowels. There may be systemic upset with pyrexia and tachycardia, and this may also lead to septicaemia. Infection may track along the portal circulation leading to portal pyaemia and a liver abscess.

A pilonidal sinus is associated with local discomfort, a moist discharge and recurrent abscess formation.

Treatment

Early drainage of an ischiorectal or perianal abscess, usually under antibiotic cover, should be undertaken and a careful examination carried out under anaesthetic lest a fistula or sinus is missed.

A pilonidal abscess should be drained surgically but, in the absence of an abscess, the track should be opened and allowed to granulate. Alternatively, the sinus should be excised fully and a primary closure obtained.

Fig. 104 An ischiorectal abscess.

Fig. 105 A recurrent pilonidal abscess. Note the pit and the purulent discharge.

Foreign bodies

Aetiology

Ingested foreign bodies may become lodged in the rectum; alternatively, they may be introduced from below during sexual activity and are usually phallic in shape. Occasionally, they may be accidental in aetiology (Fig. 106).

Clinical features

There may be features of intestinal obstruction or pain in the perineum. X-rays confirm the presence of the foreign material and exclude complications such as perforation of the bowel. Digital rectal examination should be done carefully lest the material should be pushed beyond reach.

Treatment

If introduced from above (Fig. 107), foreign material is most likely to impact in the upper oesophagus, at the pylorus or at the ileocaecal valve. If it is in the rectum, it is likely to pass spontaneously.

Foreign bodies introduced from below slip beyond the anal sphincter and into the rectum. Digital removal may be possible (Fig. 108), but this often proves difficult because of discomfort and inability to grasp the object. General anaesthesia allows full relaxation, dilatation of the anal sphincter and removal via a sigmoidoscope or colonoscope.

Fig. 106 Perianal wound resulting from impalement on a 14 cm spike.

Fig. 107 Ingested foreign bodies: spot the razor blade.

Fig. 108 Rectal foreign body removed in the A & E department.

Paraphimosis

Aetiology

The tight prepuce becomes trapped behind the engorged glans penis and each becomes further swollen (Fig. 109). The patient is usually a young adult who is reluctant to seek help and any delay in seeking treatment makes the problem worse due to venous engorgement.

Treatment

Application of an ice pack may allow the swelling to reduce sufficiently to allow reduction but an alternative is to inject hyaluronidase and local anaesthetic into the constricting band prior to reduction.

Wounds

Aetiology

Frenular tears can occur, usually during sexual intercourse. The frenal artery may be torn and this causes dramatic bleeding.

Treatment

It may be necessary to under-run and ligate the artery but it is seldom necessary to suture the wound, which heals without any problem.

Genital infections

The significance of these conditions to an A & E department is to identify them and refer them to an appropriate unit without giving treatment which might mask specialist tests. The most common infections seen are non-specific urethritis, gonorrhoea (Fig. 110) and herpetic infections (Fig. 111). This latter condition is often very painful and may lead to acute retention of urine and the patient may require admission to the hospital.

Fig. 109 A paraphimosis.

Fig. 110 Gonococcal urethritis.

Fig. 111 Herpetic vulvovaginitis.

Urethral trauma

This must be suspected whenever there has been major trauma resulting in a pelvic fracture (Fig. 112) or trauma involving the perineum. The diagnosis would be suggested by perineal or scrotal haematoma (Fig. 113), blood at the external urethral meatus or a high-riding prostate on digital rectal examination. Urethral catheterization must not be attempted and all such cases must be referred for a urological opinion (Fig. 114).

The fractured pelvis

Diagnosis

Instability or pain with pelvic springing are not reliable signs of a pelvic fracture. It should be suspected in all cases of major trauma and appropriate radiographs taken.

Treatment

Blood loss into the loose pelvic tissues and retroperitoneal space can be very substantial, so adequate intravenous fluid should be given including blood transfusion. Urgent reduction and fixation of displaced fractures should be undertaken, particularly if there is clinical evidence of continued haemorrhage. If urgent surgery is necessary and there is any delay which jeopardizes the patient's condition, a MAST suit (military anti-shock trousers) may be applied to gain time, but this should be the exception rather than the rule.

Fig. 112 Fracture–separation of the symphysis pubis and left sacroiliac joint.

Fig. 113 Perineal bruising resulting from falling astride a blunt object.

Fig. 114 Suspected urethral injury catheterized safely by a urologist.

Urine retention

Aetiology

This can present due to prostatic obstruction or blood clot from a bladder lesion such as a papilloma. More commonly, it results from blockage of an indwelling catheter (Fig. 115) in a patient referred from the community.

Clinical features

There is a painfully swollen bladder, often with overflow incontinence. 'Chronic' retention usually presents with painless bladder distension and overflow.

Treatment

Local policy will dictate whether the urologist or A & E staff performs the catheterization. Whenever it is done, it is important to use a full aseptic technique and arrange for formal review in order to diagnose and treat the underlying pathology.

Retention in women is uncommon and is usually due to a neurological disorder, pelvic obstruction by an ovarian cyst, tumour or by herpes simplex vulvitis.

Testicular torsion

This is a true emergency. The age group is between puberty and the late twenties.

Clinical features

There is acute onset of lower abdominal pain with testicular discomfort. The testis is swollen (Fig. 116) and tender and there is thickening of the vas deferens.

The differential diagnosis is from epididymo-orchitis.

Treatment

Urgent ultrasonography, followed by surgery if the diagnosis is confirmed.

Fig. 115 Long-term indwelling suprapubic catheter. Note the left inguinal hernia.

Fig. 116 Four-day-old torsion of the left testis.

Aetiology

Fracture of the femoral neck occurs most commonly in the elderly as a result of minor trauma, or in patients with porotic bones. The differential diagnosis is from a fracture of the pubic rami. Other causes include exacerbation of degenerative disease and dislocation of the hip or a prosthesis.

Clinical features

There is pain in the hip and difficulty bearing weight. The posture of the limb gives evidence of the diagnosis: a patient presenting with a fracture of the femoral neck has external rotation of the limb because of spasm in the psoas major and there is shortening of the limb (Fig. 117) whilst, in one who has dislocated the hip, there is adduction, internal rotation and flexion at the hip (Fig. 118). Active and passive movements of the hip are painful. Fracture of the pubic rami produces no abnormal posture. Pelvic springing may be painful and, if extensive or grossly displaced, the fracture may result in hypovolaemia or damage to the bladder or urethra.

X-rays of the pelvis and hip are necessary to confirm the clinical diagnosis.

Treatment

Referral for admission to hospital is usually necessary. Non-displaced fractures of the pubic rami can be treated at home with analgesia providing there is sufficient social support.

Fig. 117 Fracture of the right femoral neck.

Fig. 118 Posterior dislocation of the right hip.

Anatomy

The inguinal ligament is not a ligament in the strict sense but the lower free margin of the external oblique aponeurosis. It spans the interval between the anterior superior iliac spine and pubic tubercle. Structures passing deep to the ligament include the femoral neurovascular bundle, the musculotendinous units of psoas and iliacus and also loose connective tissue and lymphatics in the femoral canal.

Clinical relevance

The femoral artery is the key structure in the region and lies halfway between the anterior superior iliac spine and the pubic symphysis, lying medial to the mid-inguinal point. The femoral vein and nerve lie 1 cm medially and laterally respectively. The neurovascular bundle lies superficially and may be damaged easily ('butcher's thigh'—Fig. 119). Do not explore wounds in the A & E department but refer the patient to an appropriate surgeon for formal exploration in theatre.

Venous and arterial blood can be drawn easily or the vein cannulated by direct puncture or cut down on to the great saphenous vein which drains into the femoral vein just distal to the groin skin crease.

Femoral nerve block
This is of great benefit in the management of a fracture of the femoral shaft, patellar dislocation and some femoral neck fractures. The local anaesthetic solution is infiltrated in all directions around the nerve (Fig. 120) to produce profound analgesia. This obviates the need for opiates.

Fig. 119 Damage to the femoral vessels resulting from a stab wound.

Fig. 120 A femoral nerve block.

General injury

History

The mechanism of injury may give essential clues as to the likely injury but the speed of the incident is often so great that the patient cannot remember the details.

Rapid swelling of the joint (within an hour) is likely to be due to a haemarthrosis (Fig. 121). This is very painful and is due to damage to bone, or to capsular or ligamentous structures.

Swelling developing more slowly is likely to be due to synovial irritation. The swelling is not tense or particularly painful.

Investigation

Clinical examination is the most important. Plain X-rays may show the presence of an obvious fracture, but the presence of a lipohaemarthrosis (Fig. 122) is pathognomonic of an intra-articular fracture. This is seen on the lateral film with a horizontal beam as a layer of less dense fat floating on more dense blood in the suprapatellar pouch.

Treatment

A tense haemarthrosis should be aspirated under strict aseptic conditions. If done under anaesthesia, examination of the ligamentous structures can be assessed fully.

Fig. 121 A haemarthrosis in the right knee.

Fig. 122 A lipohaemarthrosis—note the horizontal fat/blood fluid level.

Ligament injuries

History

A varus or valgus force may suggest a collateral ligament injury. Paradoxically, a complete rupture produces little pain or swelling.

Clinical features

A patient with a partial tear will have pain when bearing weight, whilst a complete rupture may cause little disability if walking steadily in a straight line. Varus and valgus stability is afforded by both the collateral and cruciate ligaments. If a collateral ligament injury is suspected, the joint must be stressed in a position of 30° flexion since, in the extended position, intact cruciate ligaments can account for apparently full stability (Fig. 123).

Cruciate ligament stability is tested in a position of 90° flexion and an attempt made to draw the upper tibia forwards and backwards (Fig. 124). Instability of the anterior and posterior ligament respectively, is suggested by increased displacement compared with the normal side.

Treatment

Injuries to the ligaments require referral to an orthopaedic surgeon. Less severe injuries will be immobilized initially in a cylinder cast whilst more severe injuries may require surgical intervention.

Fig. 123 Complete rupture of the medial collateral and both cruciate ligaments.

Fig. 124 Positive posterior drawer sign due to a torn posterior cruciate ligament.

Anterior knee pain

Ruptured quadriceps

This occurs mainly in the older age group as a result of a fall.

Clinical features

There is local tenderness and a gap in the tendon is palpable just above the patella (Fig. 125). It is confirmed by the inability to extend the knee against gravity or lift the foot clear from the couch.

Treatment

Treatment is operative.

Patellar dislocation

Aetiology

The patella dislocates laterally (Fig. 126) because of the direction of action of the quadriceps muscle and the relatively shallow lateral femoral condyle. A small, high-lying patella predisposes to dislocation which occurs most commonly in young women.

Clinical features

Most patients will relocate the patella before they attend hospital so the diagnosis relies upon the history, local swelling and a positive apprehension test. This is a concerned expression and contraction of the quadriceps if the patella is subluxed laterally.

X-rays must include a skyline view to identify a marginal patellar or femoral condylar fracture.

Treatment

Treatment is conservative by immobilization in a cylinder cast following aspiration of the effusion if it is tense.

Fig. 125 Rupture of the quadriceps tendon.

Fig. 126 Lateral dislocation of the right patella.

Quadriceps wasting

Patients who have sustained an injury to the knee may rapidly develop wasting of the quadriceps muscle (Fig. 127). All such patients must be given instruction on quadriceps exercises to maintain muscle bulk since this has an important stabilizing function on both the knee and patellofemoral joints. The clinical entity of a knee which 'gives way' is due to transient loss of power in the quadriceps muscle and is a reflex phenomenon, resulting most commonly from chondromalacia patellae, entrapment of a synovial fold, a loose body or a torn meniscus.

The locked knee

Get a clear history. True locking is the terminal loss of extension (Fig. 128) and a block is firm rather than spongy.

Aetiology

There is a mechanical block due to a fragment of a torn meniscus, or a loose body, resulting from trauma or osteochondritis dissecans. The fragment floats into the joint between the femoral and tibial condyles and causes the mechanical block. The block often resolves spontaneously because the fragment floats into the suprapatellar pouch.

Treatment

A patient with a locked knee requires admission for examination under anaesthesia, followed by arthroscopy and removal of the loose fragment. Alternatively, the loose fragment can be visualized by radiography such as magnetic resonance imaging techniques.

Fig. 127 Quadriceps wasting of the right thigh associated with a knee effusion.

Fig. 128 Inability to fully extend the knee.

Varicose veins

These are dilated, tortuous subcutaneous veins which occur most commonly in the postpartum period (Fig. 129).

Clinical features

They cause aching locally and can bleed torrentially following minor trauma. Long-standing varicose veins produce distal ischaemic changes in the skin and subcutaneous tissue, particularly around the medial malleolus. Trauma may produce an ulcer which is resistant to treatment (Fig. 130).

Treatment

Haemorrhage: elevation of the limb and direct pressure over the bleeding point.

Ulcers: application of a non-adherent dressing, a firm support from toes to knee and advice regarding elevation of the limb.

Muscular pain

- Acute partial tears of the calf muscles occur most commonly in young and middle-aged adults during exertion (Fig. 131). There is local tenderness, swelling and bruising.
- A compartment syndrome following trauma or exertion results from increased pressure within one of the muscle sheaths. It produces tenderness of the muscle, pain when the muscle is stretched and, later, there is evidence of neurovascular compression.
- Spontaneous onset of calf pain raises the suspicion of a deep vein thrombosis.

Treatment

A heel raise reduces the tension in the gastrocnemius complex and elevation helps to reduce swelling of the calf muscles. A compartment syndrome should be referred to the orthopaedic surgeon. Exclude a deep venous thrombosis by investigations such as venography.

Fig. 129 Varicose veins.

Fig. 130 Varicose ulcer secondary to trauma.

Fig. 131 Partial tear of the left gastrocnemius resulting in bruising.

Ligamentous injury

Anatomy

The lateral ligament of the ankle is divided into three parts which pass forwards, downwards and backwards from the lateral malleolus. An inversion sprain causes tearing of the anterior fibres, whilst a more severe injury is associated with progressive tearing of the middle and posterior fibres which can result in instability of the joint.

Clinical features

There is marked swelling and tenderness over the lateral aspect of the ankle. Careful clinical examination does not exclude bony injury so X-rays should be taken. It is important to assess the medial aspect of the joint as well as the whole of the leg, since injuries to these areas may also occur in conjunction with an apparently isolated sprain of the lateral ligament. There may be alarming bruising which tracks along the lateral border of the foot and under the sole of the foot (Figs 132 & 133). This may itself cause an irritant synovitis of the small joints of the foot. If there is any question of ligamentous instability, stress X-rays (Fig. 134) should be performed under anaesthetic and the stability of each ankle compared.

Treatment

This is aimed at reducing the swelling and improving mobility of the ankle and subtalar complex. Rest, strapping, ice and elevation are advised and the patient is encouraged to walk as normally as possible.

Fig. 132 Swelling and bruising from a sprain of the lateral ligament.

Fig. 133 Bruising on the sole of the foot, tracking from the lateral ligament.

Fig. 134 Stress X-ray showing instability of the lateral ligament complex.

Bone and joint conditions

An extensive injury (Fig. 135) to the soft tissues or bones around the ankle may lead to dislocation or subluxation of the ankle or subtalar complex. The foot is usually displaced laterally and rotated externally relative to the leg. Reduction must be effected as a matter of urgency to prevent traction injuries to the neurovascular structures and also to minimize ischaemic damage to the skin which is under tension over the malleolus. Less extensive injuries such as fractures of the lateral malleolus (Fig. 136) are more common and often associated with sport.

Rupture of the Achilles tendon
The Achilles tendon is the combined tendinous structures of the gastrocnemius and soleus muscles. It attaches distally on to the posterior surface of the calcaneum.

Aetiology

Rupture of the Achilles tendon (Fig. 137) occurs most often in middle-aged men and results from physical exertion. The patient feels sudden pain over the tendon and this may be accompanied by an audible snap.

Clinical features

When seen early, there may be an easily palpable gap but, when seen later, the gap is indistinct because of haemorrhage and inflammatory oedema. When the calf is squeezed gently with the patient prone, the foot does not plantarflex to the same extent as the normal side (Simmond's test).

Treatment

Treatment may be conservative or operative and should be dictated by the preferences of the local orthopaedic surgeons.

Fig. 135 Compound fracture–dislocation of the ankle.

Fig. 136 Fracture of the lateral malleolus.

Fig. 137 Ruptured Achilles tendon.

21 / Bursitis

Anatomy

A bursa is a synovial sac which is a protective mechanism preventing damage to soft tissues by pressure on a bony surface. Bursae occur typically over bony prominences but may occur also in relation to tendons or ligaments at major joints (Figs 138 & 139).

Aetiology

Inflammation is most commonly sterile and related to a repetitive occupational activity (Fig. 140). Occasionally, the bursitis may be infective and associated with an abrasion or an episode of septicaemia. Rarely, the bursitis may be gouty or rheumatoid in origin.

Clinical features

The area shows the cardinal features of acute inflammation, heat, redness, pain and loss of movement and there may also be crepitus. There is usually no associated lymphatic involvement and aspiration of the bursa reveals pale yellow serous fluid. Infective, gouty or rheumatoid bursitis is associated with turbid, thick aspirate and laboratory examination of the fluid may be very helpful in confirming the diagnosis.

Treatment

Sterile bursitis is treated by rest, support, local ice pack and non-steroidal anti-inflammatory agents. If non-infective bursitis has not responded to this treatment, it may be treated by aspiration and instillation of a locally acting steroid. Infective bursitis should be drained surgically and the other unusual causes should be treated by a rheumatologist.

Fig. 138 An olecranon bursa.

Fig. 139 Prepatellar bursa (housemaid's knee).

Fig. 140 Occupational bursitis in a tailor.

Virus infections

Herpes zoster

This is due to varicella zoster virus which emerges from posterior roots of the spinal nerves and the sensory cranial nerves.

Clinical features

There is prodromal pain which can mimic visceral pain such as a myocardial infarction. After a few days, redness of the skin develops and vesicles appear within a particular dermatome (Fig. 141).

Treatment

Acyclovir may be used to treat the skin lesions. Sufficiently strong analgesia is important.

Herpes simplex

Clinical features

This is subdivided into type I, which is associated predominantly with oral lesions (cold sores), and type II, which is associated predominantly with genital lesions, but this rule is not always true. Occasionally, the virus can affect the corneal epithelium to produce a dendritic ulcer (see also Fig. 37, p. 30 & Fig. 111, p. 84).

Treatment

Early treatment with acyclovir ointment can reduce the severity of the lesions.

Warts

Clinical features

These are common and found mainly on the hands (Fig. 142). They are spread by direct contact and may be painful if present on the feet.

Treatment

Treatment may be by topical salicylic acid or cryotherapy with liquid nitrogen.

Molluscum contagiosum

Clinical features

An unusual condition which presents with clusters of painless, discrete, pearly, raised lesions without any surrounding erythema (Fig. 143).

Treatment

Treatment is by pricking the centre of each with a sharpened wooden stick which has been dipped in phenol solution or betadine.

Fig. 141 Herpes zoster.

Fig. 142 Warts.

Fig. 143 Molluscum contagiosum.

Miscellaneous conditions

Eczema

Aetiology

This is usually allergic in nature but may also be due to atopy. Allergic eczema may be due to medication, plants, animals or cosmetics. Jewellery, particularly items containing nickel, produces characteristic patterns of eczema (Fig. 144).

Clinical features

Eczema presents as an itchy rash which forms vesicles and these break down and become encrusted.

Treatment

Referral to a dermatologist should be made in order to identify any definite allergens and to advise about prevention of further problems.

Topical steroids are used. Care must be taken regarding the strength of the steroid, particularly if they are used on the face, as skin atrophy and telangiectasia can result. If there is a superadded infection, a topical antibiotic may be used in conjunction with the steroid.

Pityriasis rosea

This can be an alarming rash with a 'herald patch' (Fig. 145) which is the first sign of the rash to appear. It is large, oval and has a scaly margin. Subsequently, further smaller lesions develop and these tend to be arranged in a horizontal line. The rash is self-limiting over a period of between 4 and 6 weeks.

Lichen planus

The patient may present with flat-topped, multiangular lesions which are shiny and violaceous. They are common on the flexor aspect of the wrists and may be itchy. White striations are seen on the buccal mucosa (Fig. 146).

Fig. 144 Allergy to a nickel bracelet.

Fig. 145 Herald patch in pityriasis rosea.

Fig. 146 Buccal mucosa in lichen planus.

Tumours

It is important to identify those lesions which may be readily removed without risk and to be able to identify those lesions which should be referred to a dermatologist as they may be malignant.

Clinical types

Melanoma.   This is usually a dark, pigmented lesion with an irregular border. There may be the history of a pre-existing mole which has increased recently in size, may have bled, ulcerated or become itchy. Beware of the subungual melanoma (Fig. 147) which may inadvertently be explored as an infection or haematoma.

Rodent ulcer.   This is a basal cell carcinoma which occurs most commonly on the face (Fig. 148). It has a raised, shiny edge and dilated blood vessels may cross this edge. Although it does not metastasize, it is locally very invasive.

Squamous cell carcinoma.   This is a hard nodule which may appear warty (Fig. 149). Larger lesions ulcerate and metastasis is not uncommon. Treatment is by local excision or radiotherapy.

Keratoacanthoma.   This is a rapidly growing, benign skin tumour which may ulcerate (Fig. 150). It may resemble a squamous cell carcinoma histologically, but the rapid growth and spontaneous resolution are pathognomonic.

Fig. 147 Subungual melanoma.

Fig. 148 Locally invasive rodent ulcer.

Fig. 149 A squamous cell carcinoma presenting as a wart.

Fig. 150 A keratoacanthoma.

Aetiology

Cellulitis (Fig. 151): a rapidly spreading infection of subcutaneous tissue caused most often by *Streptococcus pyogenes*. It may be haematogenous or introduced by an apparently insignificant wound.

Pyogenic infection: may develop de novo or in a pre-existing cyst (Fig. 152). The most common organism is *Staphylococcus aureus* and an abscess may develop anywhere but the most common sites are the breast, axilla and ischiorectal fossa.

Clinical features

Cellulitis produces an area which is red, warm, tender and swollen and there may be features of systemic upset with fever and tachycardia. In addition, a pyogenic infection presents a localized fluctuant swelling.

Treatment

Cellulitis: treated with high dose antibiotics and the patient reviewed daily. If systemic upset is a prominent feature, admission to hospital is advised and intravenous antibiotics given.

Pyogenic infection: the abscess can be treated by opening with a cruciate incision and trimming off the corners (Fig. 153). This ensures that the skin wound does not heal before the cavity becomes obliterated with granulation tissue. Alternatively, the cavity can be curetted and packed loosely with paraffin gauze or obliterated with large mattress sutures. If the latter is undertaken, a loading dose of antibiotic is given preoperatively or antibiotic cream may be injected into the cavity.

Fig. 151 Cellulitis with lymphangitis—the 'red lines of death'.

Fig. 152 Infected sebaceous cyst.

Fig. 153 Cruciate incision to treat an abscess on the buttock.

Pyogenic granuloma

This is a small nodule of granulation tissue which occurs most commonly on the fingers following minor trauma. It grows slowly and there is no associated cellulitis.

Treatment

Thorough curettage should be performed and the specimen sent for histological confirmation. Small recurrences may be cauterized with silver nitrate or liquid nitrogen (Fig. 154).

Paronychia

An infection of the nail fold may track proximally beneath the cuticle or the nail (Fig. 155).

Treatment

Early treatment with antibiotics may prevent the formation of pus but it often requires drainage over the area of maximum fluctuation or by opening the interval between the nail and cuticle. If the nail is floating freely, it should be removed completely.

Ingrowing toenails

These occur commonly in adolescent or young adult males and affect the nail folds (Fig. 156).

Treatment

Conservative treatment may effect a temporary cure but surgical intervention is usually required. A wide variety of surgical procedures are used with variable results and it is recognized that simple nail avulsion leads to an unacceptably high recurrence rate. Wedge resection of the nail followed by ablation of the germinal matrix with liquified phenol is a simple and effective cure with a low recurrence rate.

Fig. 154 Recurrence of pyogenic granuloma treated with silver nitrate.

Fig. 155 A paronychia.

Fig. 156 An ingrowing toenail.

Unusual conditions

Erysipelas
Erysipelas (Fig. 157) is a streptococcal infection of skin and subcutaneous tissue.

Clinical features

The lesion is sharply demarcated and has a palpable edge. The face is most commonly affected and there may be associated systemic upset requiring hospital admission.

Treatment

Treatment is with oral or intramuscular penicillin.

Orf
Orf (Fig. 158) is an infection of the skin of viral aetiology. It occurs commonly on the hands of those working with sheep.

Clinical features

It presents with a localized, painless maculopapular rash which vesiculates. This may then break down, become painful and secondarily infected.

Treatment

Treatment is with topical idoxuridine with appropriate systemic antibiotics if secondary infection has developed. It should not be drained surgically despite its appearance.

Anthrax
Anthrax (Fig. 159) is a now rare bacterial infection which also occurs predominantly in farmers and in those workers who handle animal skins.

Clinical features

It produces a pruritic red papule which vesiculates and progresses to a painless black eschar with marked surrounding non-pitting oedema. There may be systemic upset.

Treatment

Treatment is with regular intramuscular penicillin.

Fig. 157 Erysipelas requiring hospitalization.

Fig. 158 Orf.

Fig. 159 The black eschar of anthrax.

Aetiology

These are due to corrosive chemicals, heat, electricity or some other high energy source. The damage to the skin and deeper tissues depends upon the duration of contact and the temperature or energies involved.

Scalds

Scalds occur from hot liquid or steam, and are usually superficial. They are moist, red, blistered and exquisitely painful as the nerve endings are intact (Fig. 160).

Treatment

These are treated conservatively by dressing with non-adherent dressings and they heal spontaneously within 14 days. Extensive blisters (Fig. 161) should not be deroofed as this leaves a very sensitive area—just aspirate and dress.

Deep burns

The full extent may take some days to become apparent. They develop slough on the burned area and sensation is impaired. Full-thickness burns are charred (Fig. 162), the skin is anaesthetic due to destruction of nerve endings and feels firm.

Treatment

Surgical débridement followed by skin grafting is required.

Inhalation injury

Facial burns are usually superficial and, because of the good blood supply, heal very quickly. They are treated by exposure rather than by dressing. Alarming swelling may develop within the first 48 h and this can impair the airway, particularly if there has been inhalation of smoke or other hot gas (Fig. 163). Look for singeing of nasal hair and the presence of intra-oral soot. If in doubt, contact an anaesthetist with a view to early intubation to protect the airway.

Fig. 160 A scald from hot water.

Fig. 161 A large blister on a hand.

Fig. 162 Fatal deep burns.

Fig. 163 Inhalation damage to the airway.

Chemical burns

These usually occur in accidents in laboratories or industrial plants but may occasionally be self-inflicted (Fig. 164). They often involve acids or alkalis but may also involve a variety of organic chemicals.

Treatment

Treatment is by washing the area liberally with running water. Some specific antidotes exist, such as topical calcium gluconate gel or calcium gluconate injection locally for hydrofluoric acid, and topical sodium bicarbonate solution for acid burns. Burns with alkali are more serious than with acid because the alkali penetrates the skin and continues to burn the subcutaneous tissue, resulting in a deeper burn than is first anticipated. A little-appreciated problem is that cement is alkaline and may cause extensive burns of the legs and feet (Fig. 165) if spillage over the top of boots is not recognized and treated immediately.

Hand burns

These usually result in marked swelling.

Treatment

Superficial burns are treated conservatively by elevation and application of silver sulphadiazine cream, followed by enclosure of the hand in a loosely fitting plastic bag. This is to minimize swelling and encourage active mobilization of the fingers from the earliest possible time. This can result in a rather alarming appearance (Fig. 166) which needs to be explained to the patient.

Fig. 164 Self-inflicted burns with acid to destroy a tattoo.

Fig. 165 'Wellington boot' cement burn. Note the line of the sock.

Fig. 166 Burn of the hand treated with a large glove and silver sulphadiazine.

25 / Wound care

General

Wounds may be incised by a sharp object, or be lacerated with irregular edges and made by a blunt object or by tearing the skin. Always elicit an accurate history of the aetiology so as to be aware of possible complications or forensic connotations. Beware of a stab wound as the size of the skin wound bears little relation to the depth and direction of the wound track.

Closure

Most wounds can be closed by suture. Adhesive tapes (Fig. 167) can be used in superficial wounds and obviate the need for local anaesthesia. This is of particular value in children. Histoacryl skin cement is used occasionally, particularly to close scalp wounds.

Problems

Wounds more than 8 h old are likely to be contaminated. They should be cleaned thoroughly, left open and considered for secondary suture after a period of 3 or 4 days. This reduces the risk of infection and subsequent wound breakdown.

A knuckle wound (Fig. 168) which has resulted from a blow to a victim's mouth may have produced tendon and joint capsular injuries. These are not obvious if the finger is examined with the finger extended. They require antibiotic cover and careful review.

If a wound looks as if it needs another suture, it probably does. If it looks as if it has been sutured too tightly, it has and will result in tissue necrosis (Fig. 169). ➡

Fig. 167 Facial sutures and adhesive tapes.

Fig. 168 A 4-day-old punch wound is best left open.

Fig. 169 Wound breakdown produced by suturing too tightly.

All wounds must be explored thoroughly under local or general anaesthetic. If bleeding cannot be controlled by direct pressure, a tourniquet can be applied for a short period. When exploring a wound, first exclude the presence of foreign material. If some is found, check that there is no more. Consider carefully each structure in the area of the wound and check its integrity, even if clinical examination shows apparently full function of neurovascular and tendinous structures. Nerve injuries in the hand or proximal parts of the fingers warrant careful surgical repair.

Cut tendons can be missed easily (Figs 170 & 171). Initially there may be a partial division which may progress subsequently to a complete rupture, particularly when the initial discomfort has subsided and the patient uses the limb normally. Alternatively, when examined clinically, the patient may be in too much pain to move the limb properly and so a divided tendon may be suspected when this is not the case.

Fig. 170 Cut flexor tendon to the ring finger.

Fig. 171 Cut tibialis anterior tendon from glass.

Pretibial wounds

Clinical features

These do not heal very well in any age group but healing is particularly slow in postmenopausal women. The subcutaneous tissue is thin and the skin is friable. There is often a flap of tissue which rolls back like a roller blind and so the surface epithelium is in contact with the subcutaneous tissue and does not heal (Fig. 172).

Treatment

The flap should be cleaned thoroughly and replaced gently to its normal position. It may be held in place by the sparing use of absorbable subcutaneous sutures or the use of steristrips. More recently, Histoacryl glue has been used to anchor the fragile skin edges with success. The skin should not be sutured as this results in necrosis of the flap (Fig. 173). Alternatively, the flap may be 'de-fatted' and used as a fenestrated in situ graft, being held with a few, lightly tied sutures (Figs 174 & 175). This gives valuable cover to a potentially extensive wound. The patient must rest with the leg elevated, but active mobilization around the house is advised towards the end of the first week.

The wound is dressed with a non-adherent dressing such as tulle-gras or Viscopaste. The wound may break down to form an ulcer which requires dressings until healing has occurred and this may take 12 weeks.

Fig. 172 Bilateral pretibial lacerations. Note the roller blind edge on the left leg.

Fig. 173 Necrotic flap resulting from suturing.

Fig. 174 Large pretibial wound with the base of the flap intact.

Fig. 175 A fenestrated in situ graft using the flap.

Pretibial haematoma

This is very painful due to the tense swelling. There is a tendency for the skin over the haematoma to necrose because of the pressure (Fig. 176).

Treatment

Ideally, the haematoma should be drained before necrosis occurs. Aspiration is associated with recurrence so the skin should be incised and a surprisingly large volume of coagulated blood will be evacuated. If skin necrosis has occurred, this must be removed (Fig. 177). The wound should be packed lightly with non-adherent material and a firm dressing applied. Further treatment is as for a pretibial laceration.

Dog bites

Treatment

The wound should be cleaned thoroughly, and wounds on the face (Fig. 178) may be closed carefully to produce a good cosmetic result. Extensive wounds elsewhere may also be closed, but it is important that suturing should be done lightly to allow escape of any exudate which may collect. Small wounds are cleaned thoroughly and left open. Do not forget to check the tetanus immunity of the patient and consider antibiotics, particularly if the wound is old or signs of infection are present at first consultation.

Fish hooks

Treatment

Under local anaesthetic, push the barb through the skin in the same direction as its entry (Fig. 179). Cut the hook with wire cutters and remove it.

Fig. 176 Pretibial haematoma with skin necrosis.

Fig. 177 Necrotic skin with evacuated haematoma.

Fig. 178 Dog bite to the face.

Fig. 179 Fish hook in the finger.

26 / Foreign bodies

Aetiology

Foreign bodies in the limbs are usually due to injuries from glass or falling on to fragmented material. Wooden foreign bodies occur less commonly and are usually due to gardening accidents. Foreign bodies in the head, neck or trunk are likely to result from a missile (Fig. 180) or an assault.

Clinical features

It is important to examine neurovascular and tendinous function of a limb distal to the wound. Glass and metal are radio-opaque and an X-ray is mandatory. A wooden foreign body will not necessarily show on X-ray unless there is any associated paint on the wood or air outlines the fragment.

Localization of the foreign body by radiography involves two X-rays at right angles (Fig. 181). Metallic skin markers should be used since they give a guide to the direction and depth of the foreign material in relation to the markers whose outline should be drawn on the skin over the entry wound (Fig. 182).

Treatment

Foreign bodies are notoriously difficult to remove, even under ideal operating conditions which include general anaesthesia, a bloodless field and an operating theatre.

Foreign bodies in the chest or abdomen must be suspected of having damaged deeper structures. Intravenous access must be established and resuscitation undertaken as appropriate before referral to a surgeon for formal exploration.

Fig. 180 Air gun pellet wound to the right eye.

Fig. 181 Anteroposterior and lateral films of a needle in the great toe.

Fig. 182 Pieces of paper clip used as skin markers.

If appropriately trained plaster room staff are not available 24 h a day, A & E staff should familiarize themselves with the basic techniques to stabilize a fracture until a definitive cast can be applied. The aims are to prevent displacement at the fracture site and to preserve both the blood and nerve supplies to the limb.

Materials

Several casting materials are available. Traditionally, calcium sulphate (plaster of Paris) impregnated bandages are used and these are easy to apply either in bandage or plaster slab form.

Resin materials are lighter and more comfortable for the patient but demand much more experience to apply correctly.

Common casts

A & E staff should be competent in the application of common casts such as a back slab (Fig. 183), a scaphoid (Fig. 184) and a below knee cast (Fig. 185). It is more comfortable for the patient to have an injured limb immobilized with a cast or back slab than to use a bulky 'wool and crêpe' bandage which is likely to slip.

Technique

A layer of protective material is applied to the limb prior to the casting material to protect the underlying skin. In general, the fracture site is immobilized as well as the joints above and below the site of injury. The limb is immobilized in a position of function whenever possible but there are notable exceptions such as a Smith's fracture which is immobilized with the wrist in full dorsiflexion.

Fig. 183 A forearm back slab being applied.

Fig. 184 A scaphoid cast immobilizes the thumb.

Fig. 185 A below-knee resin cast with a walking heel.

Complications

Swelling

During the early period following an injury, there may be little bruising and swelling. This increases over the first 72 h so any cast should be well padded to allow for this swelling. A patient who returns complaining of any swelling (Fig. 186), and has clinical evidence of neurovascular compression, must have the cast split longitudinally or removed (Fig. 187). If split, it must be split down to skin since the padding material beneath the cast may also compromise the circulation.

Pressure sores

Moulding the cast by pressing the fingers on the wet cast will cause friction between the cast and skin and may result in blister formation which will break down and may become infected or necrose. A patient must be discouraged from inserting anything between the cast and skin (Fig. 188) because this also can lead to a pressure sore.

If a patient complains of increased pain at the site of an injury beneath the cast, a window should be cut in the cast to allow the underlying skin to be inspected. If the skin has not broken down, the cast can be restored and a further layer of cast material used to hold the window in place. If there is evidence of skin ischaemia or necrosis, specific treatment can be given and the window replaced temporarily, allowing daily inspection of the skin.

Fig. 186 Swelling of the hand distal to a scaphoid cast.

Fig. 187 The same hand (Fig. 186) after removal of the cast.

Fig. 188 Source of irritation and skin necrosis—the end off a knitting needle!

Gunshot wounds

Features

Gunshot wounds are divided into high velocity from rifles and low velocity from hand guns. High velocity wounds are most common in a war or terrorist situation. They are associated with massive tissue damage and are characterized by a small entry and a large exit wound. Low velocity wounds are associated with damage confined to structures in the bullet's path (Fig. 189). The bullet may follow tissue planes and remain in the patient at some distance from its expected position. Check that the number of wounds correlates with the number of bullets seen on X-ray (Fig. 190).

Treatment

This depends upon the nature and position of the wound. Try to determine the entry and exit points and the possible course followed by the bullet. Resuscitation and surgical exploration are indicated.

Bomb blasts

Features

The injuries produced depend upon the size of the explosion, whether it was in an enclosed space and the distance between it and the patient. Injuries result from the blast wave and flash as well as fragments of masonry or metal energized by the blast (Fig. 191).

Treatment

Careful assessment, resuscitation and awareness of possible pressure damage to the ear and lung.

Fig. 189 Entry and exit wounds in a hand holding a bottle.

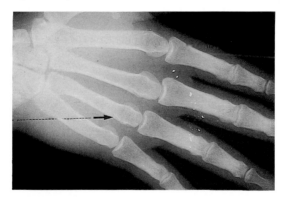

Fig. 190 Line of bullet. The foreign bodies are glass, and not bullet fragments.

Fig. 191 Flash and shrapnel wounds from a bomb explosion.

Diagnosis

The greatest care must be taken to neither miss nor misdiagnose these injuries. It takes time and experience to differentiate an accidental from a non-accidental injury (Fig. 192) so senior colleagues, who have specific experience in this field, should be consulted.

Clinical features

Factors which may alert the attending doctor to the problem include:
- the patient is already identified on the 'at risk' register
- the patient might be a frequent attender at the A & E department
- the parents or guardians give a variable history which does not fit the clinical signs (Fig. 193)
- there may be an unusual distribution of injury with an unusual appearance, such as bruising well away from bony prominences (Fig. 194)
- there may be radiological evidence of old, multiple bony injuries
- the child has a wary, worried expression and does not interact normally with other children or experienced staff on the ward.

Fig. 192 Human bite marks on the distal forearm and hand.

Fig. 193 'Bath dipping'—typically the scalds are on the buttocks and feet.

Fig. 194 Bruising of the buttocks from being beaten with a wooden stick.

Self-inflicted wounds

Repeated superficial lacerations on accessible parts of the body (Fig. 195) are often more a cry for help than an attempt at suicide. The wound may require surgical treatment but consider the whole patient as the wound is only a small part of the problem. The patient's psychological state must be assessed and, if indicated, the help of a psychiatrist should be enlisted. Follow-up must be arranged via the general practitioner if the patient is registered, but avoid situations where there may be a long delay in such follow-up.

Delivery in A & E

Occasionally a mother will give sudden and unexpected birth whilst in the department (Fig. 196). The mother is usually young, single and will have concealed the fact that she is pregnant. She will not have had any antenatal care. Share in the joy of a healthy delivery and ensure that there is both social and obstetric follow-up.

Iatrogenic problems

Treatment sometimes causes problems. One of the most common is a reaction to a tetanus toxoid injection (Fig. 197). This produces swelling and erythema as well as local pain. The patient should be reassured, treated symptomatically and followed up until the problem has settled.

Fig. 195 Self-inflicted lacerations to the wrist and forearm.

Fig. 196 Delivery in the A & E department.

Fig. 197 Reaction to tetanus toxoid.

Protect yourself

It is essential that members of staff always take precautions against contamination from patients' body fluids. Patients seen in an A & E department are mostly unknown to staff and, in situations such as major trauma or unconsciousness from alcohol or drugs, no history will be available. Assume that all patients are an infection hazard and be sure to wear gloves as the minimum protection (Fig. 198) whenever you are carrying out any invasive procedure such as venepuncture, cannulation or endotracheal intubation. Gloves must also be worn when dealing with an open wound.

High risk

If there is a case of a known HIV or hepatitis positive patient (Fig. 199), senior medical staff should be involved and full protective measures taken as appropriate, which may include the use of gowns, an apron, mask, visor and double gloves.

Low risk

Do not forget the less melodramatic infection hazards of an A & E department such as fleas, lice and scabies (Fig. 200). They are still very common, particularly in homeless individuals. Medical and nursing staff probably remain the greatest hazard to themselves and to other members of the hospital staff due to carelessness. Ensure that you personally dispose of all needles and sharps in a safe manner.

Fig. 198 A patient with Hepatitis B—note that the doctor is wearing gloves.

Fig. 199 Intravenous drug abuse.

Fig. 200 Common site of burrows in scabies

Index